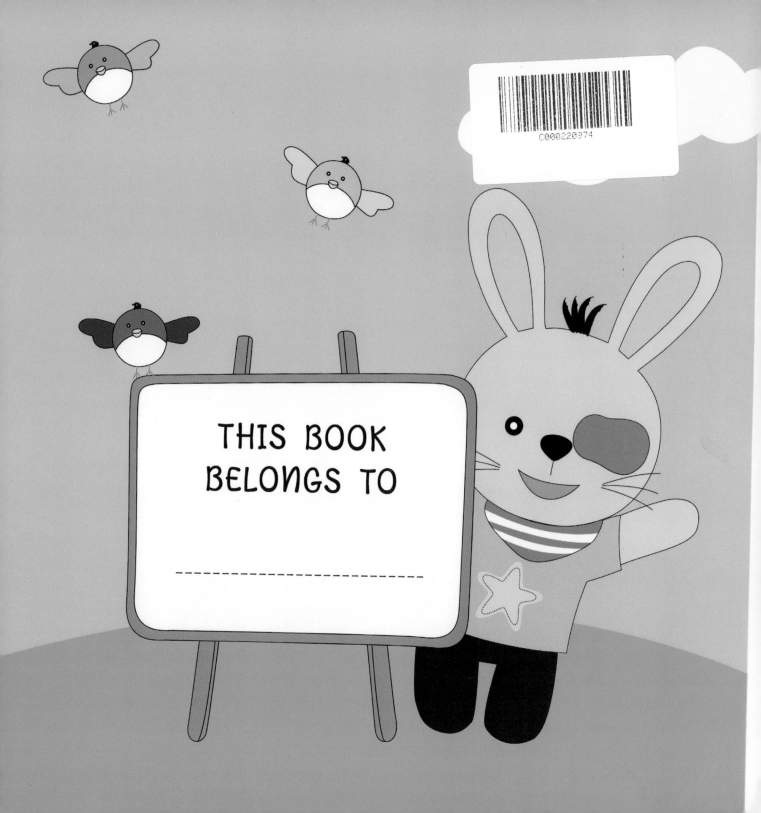

THIS BOOK
BELONGS TO

_____

C000220974

For Albert Duong

and all children
who require patching

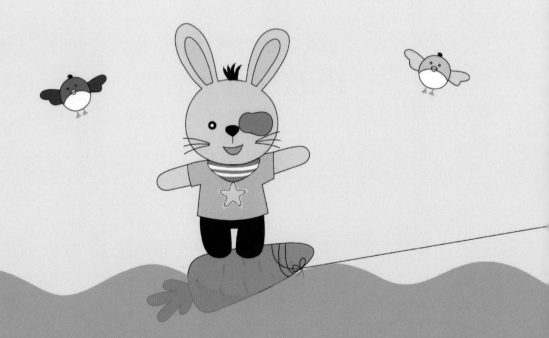

RABBIT'S SPECIAL EYES

Authors: Kathy Thach & Amanda Duong
Illustrator: Kathy Thach

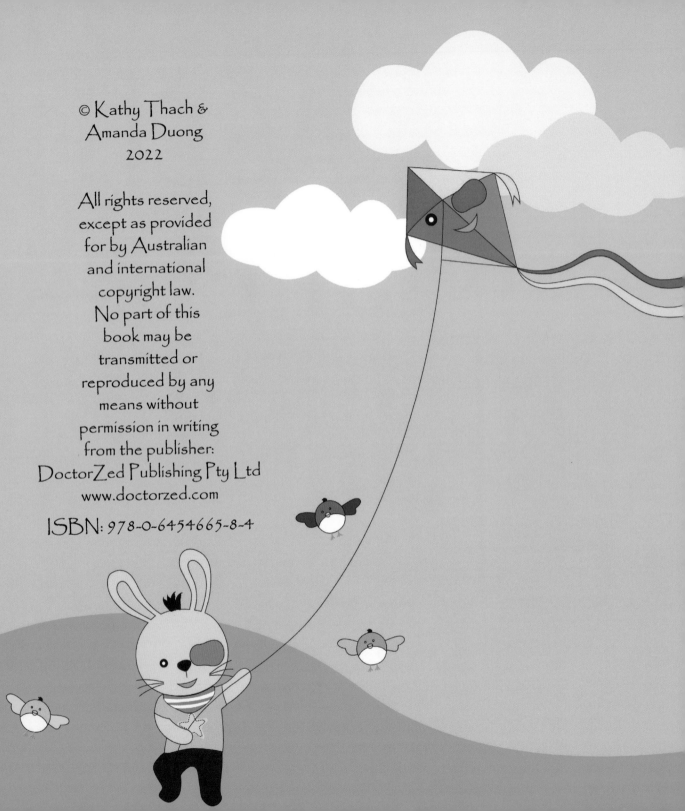

DoctorZed Publishing Pty Ltd
www.doctorzed.com

ISBN: 978-0-6454665-8-4

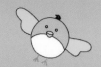

The rabbit family was
very HAPPY to welcome
a newborn baby.
He was very SWEET.
All the birds sang,
"Tweet, tweet, tweet!"

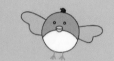

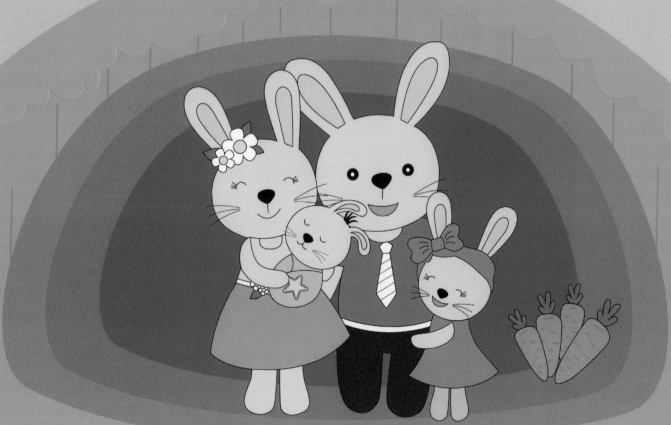

1

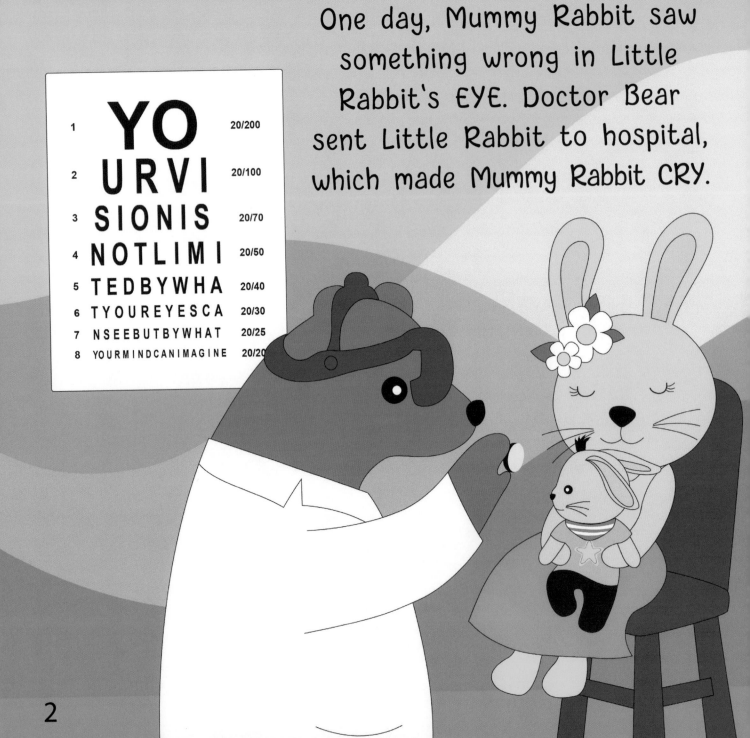

One day, Mummy Rabbit saw something wrong in Little Rabbit's EYE. Doctor Bear sent Little Rabbit to hospital, which made Mummy Rabbit CRY.

1	YO	20/200
2	URVI	20/100
3	SIONIS	20/70
4	NOTLIMI	20/50
5	TEDBYWHA	20/40
6	TYOUREYESCA	20/30
7	NSEEBUTBYWHAT	20/25
8	YOURMINDCANIMAGINE	20/20

2

After hospital,
Little Rabbit wore
a CONTACT LENS
and he could
see again.

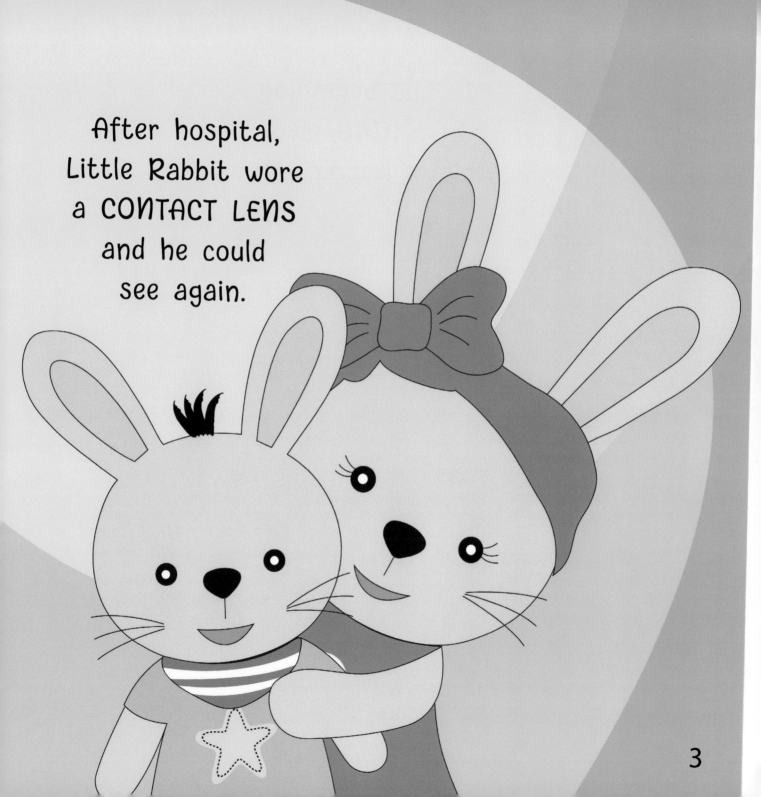

In the beginning,
PATCHING made
Little Rabbit cry.

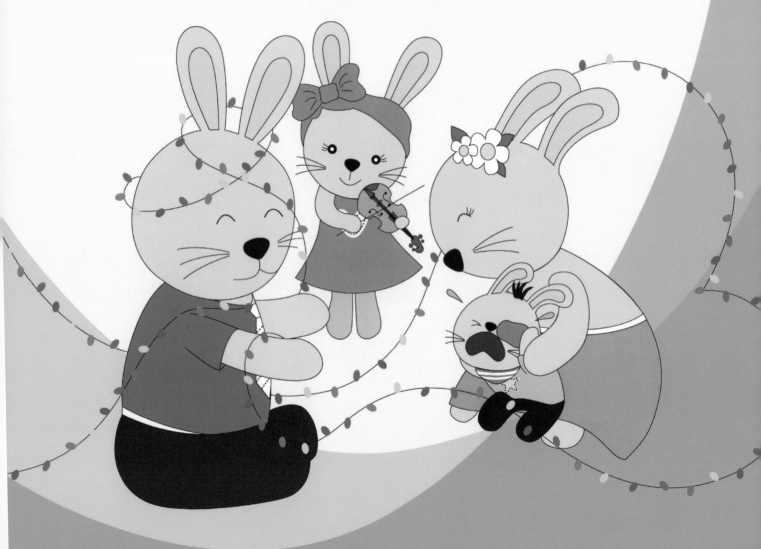

4

But soon Little Rabbit began to SMILE.

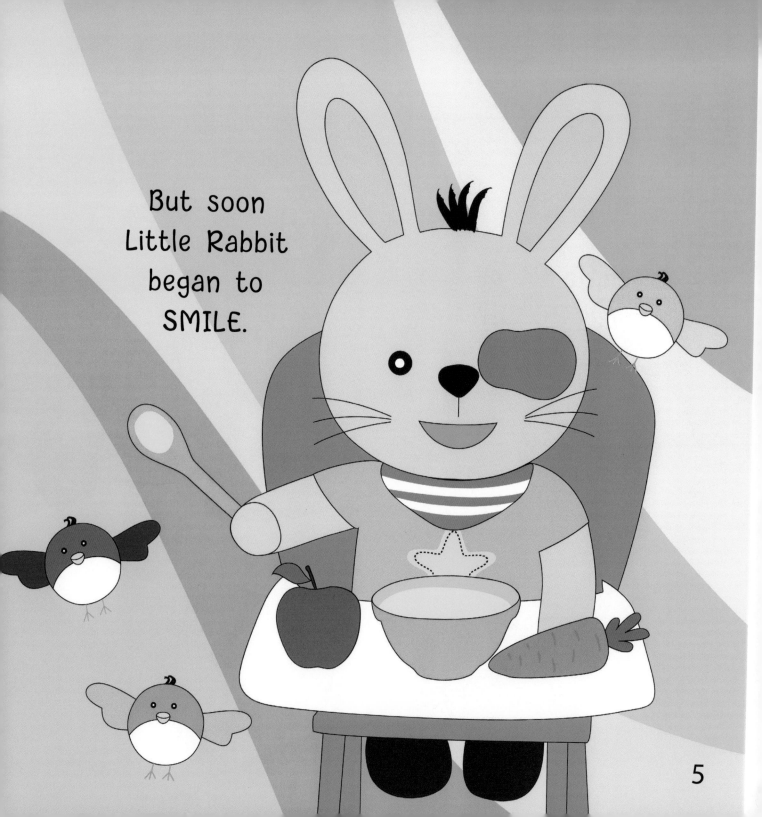

5

Little Rabbit
loved READING
while patching.

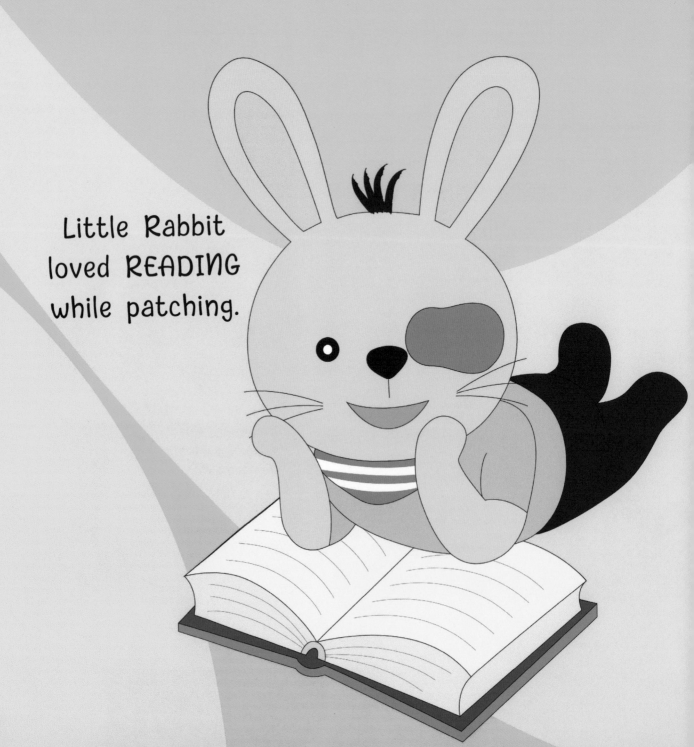

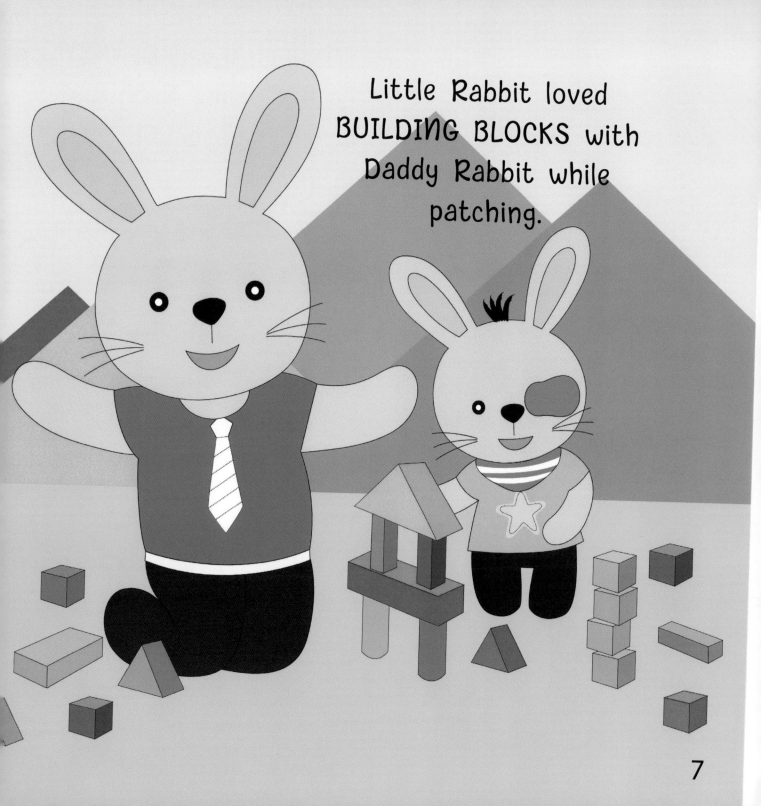

Little Rabbit loved BUILDING BLOCKS with Daddy Rabbit while patching.

Little Rabbit loved DANCING
with Mummy Rabbit
while patching.

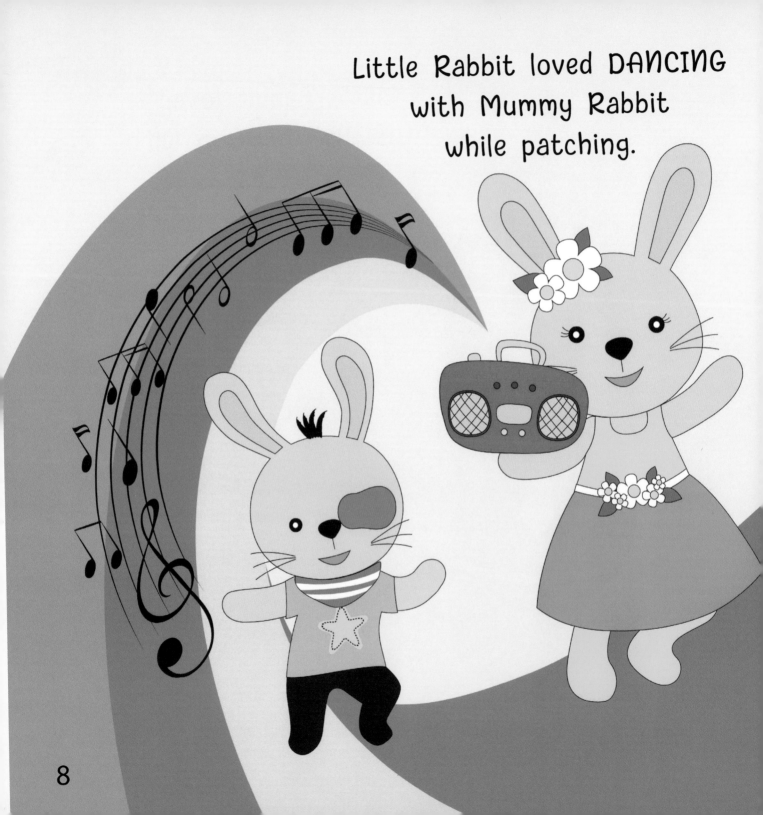

Little Rabbit loved
PLAYING hide and seek
with Sister Rabbit
while patching.

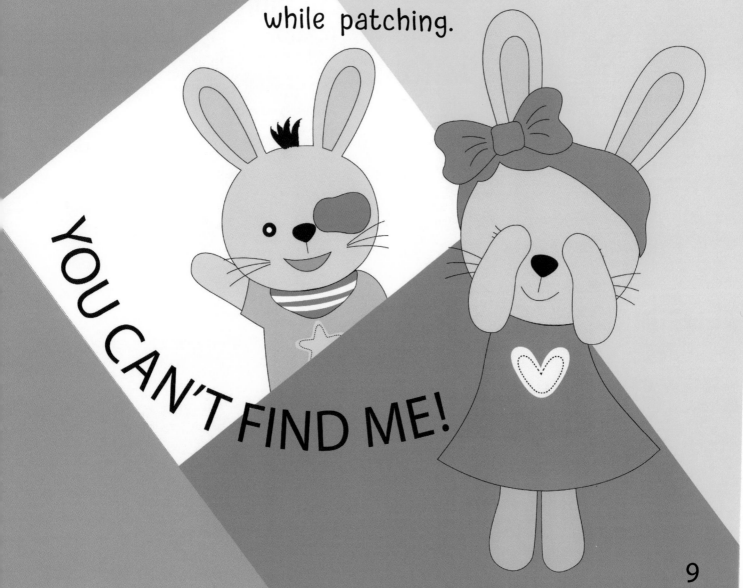

YOU CAN'T FIND ME!

Little Rabbit loved PLAYING
PIRATE GAMES while patching.
He was always a great
CAPTAIN.

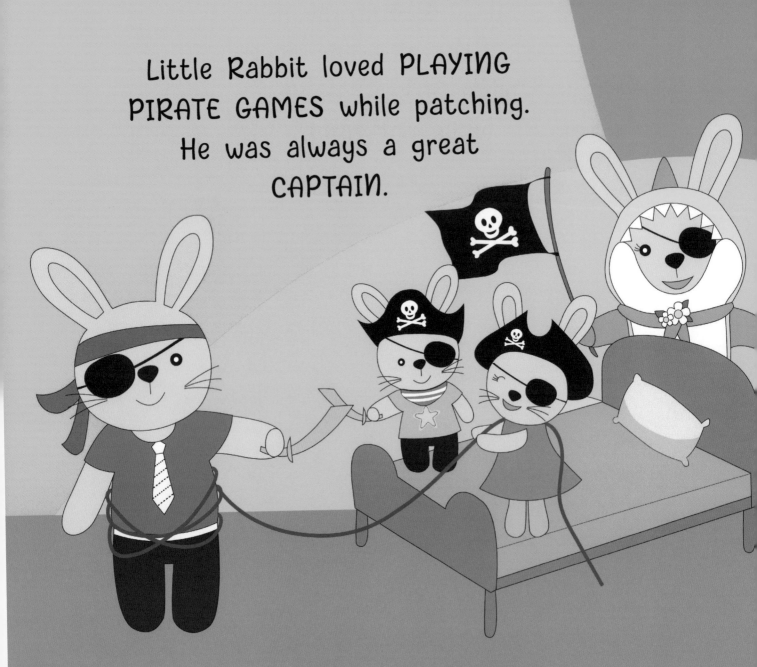

One day, while at the playground, other kids made fun of Little Rabbit.

"Why do you need a patch? You look silly!"

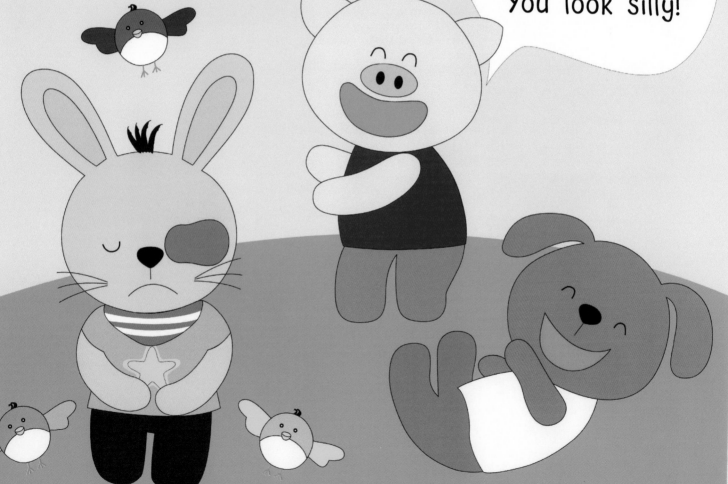

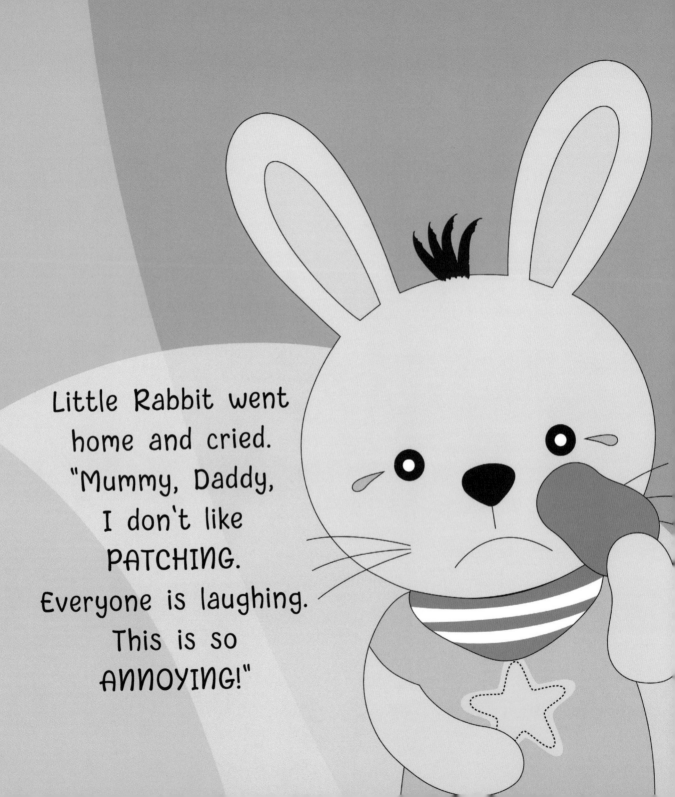

Little Rabbit went
home and cried.
"Mummy, Daddy,
I don't like
PATCHING.
Everyone is laughing.
This is so
ANNOYING!"

Mummy Rabbit and Daddy Rabbit
gave Little Rabbit a big HUG.

"Let's wipe away
your TEARS,"
said Mummy Rabbit.

"The cataract made
your eye all foggy,
just like this misty
window here,"
said Daddy Rabbit.

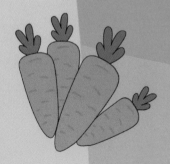

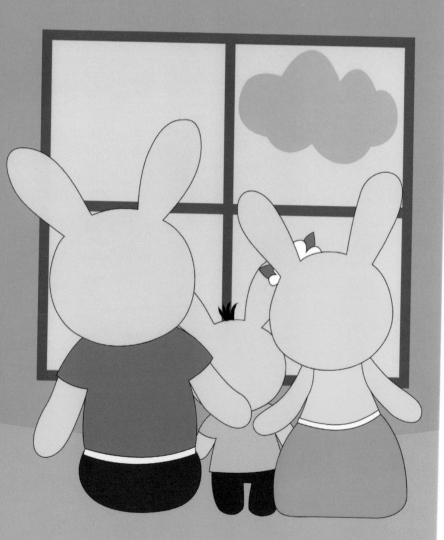

"To bring back your VISION, patching needs to be done," said Mummy Rabbit. "Your future is as bright as the sun. So don't you worry, just start having FUN."

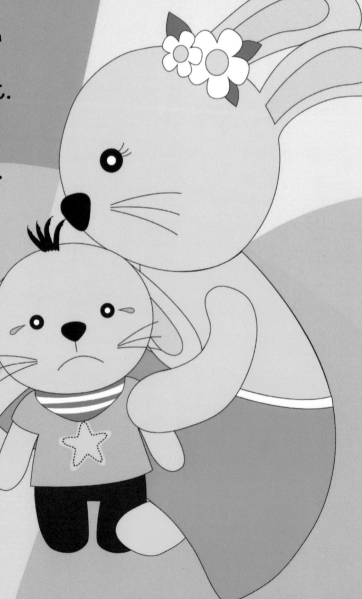

But Little Rabbit was still worried. "Will my eyes ever get BETTER? When can I stop patching?"

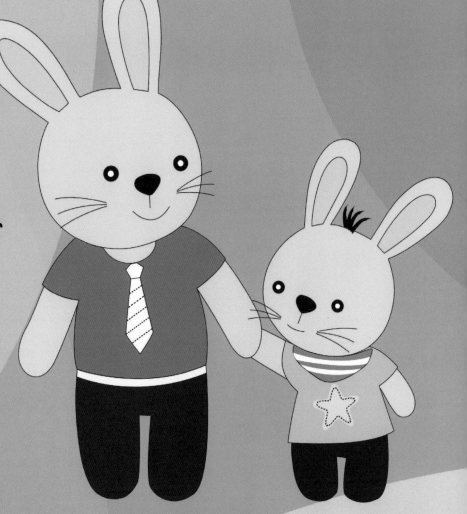

"Very soon," said Daddy Rabbit. "Just keep giving your eyes GOOD CARE."

Little Rabbit felt better.
Patching was very
important.
And he became more
CONFIDENT.

"Patching will
make my eyes
STRONGER!"

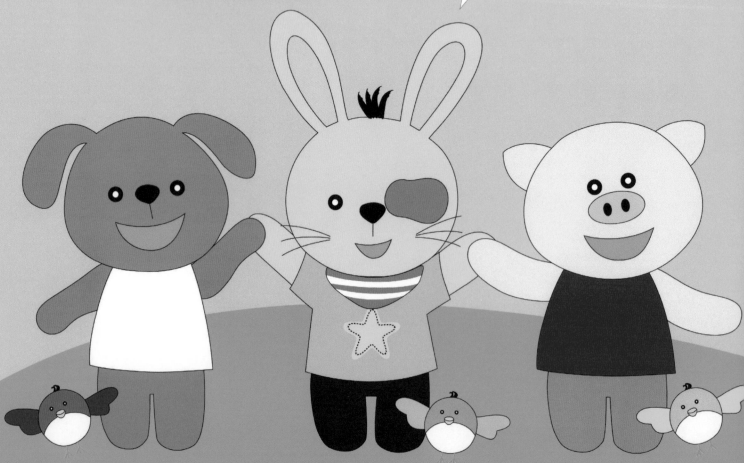

16

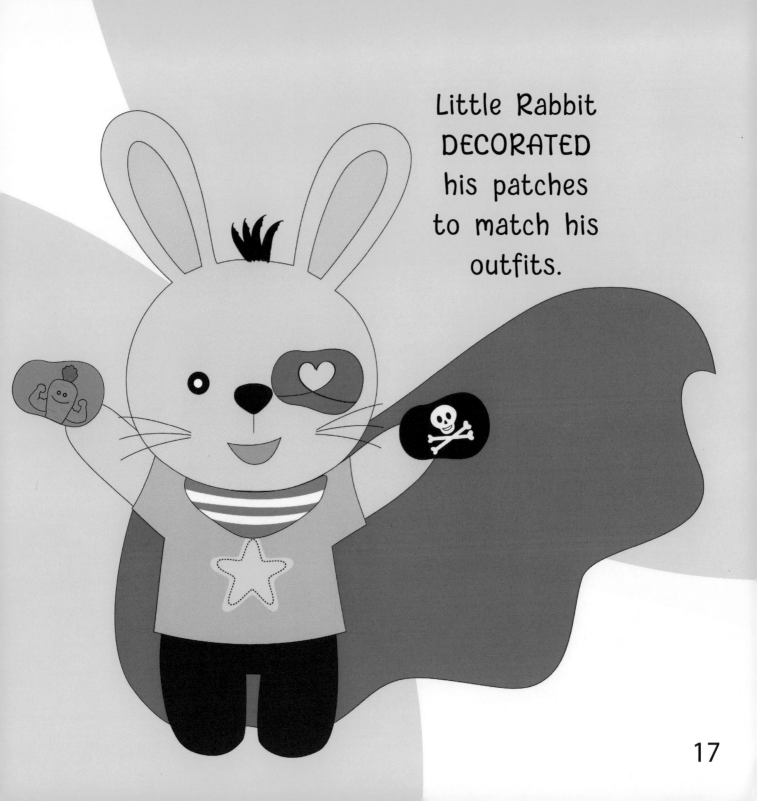

Little Rabbit
DECORATED
his patches
to match his
outfits.

17

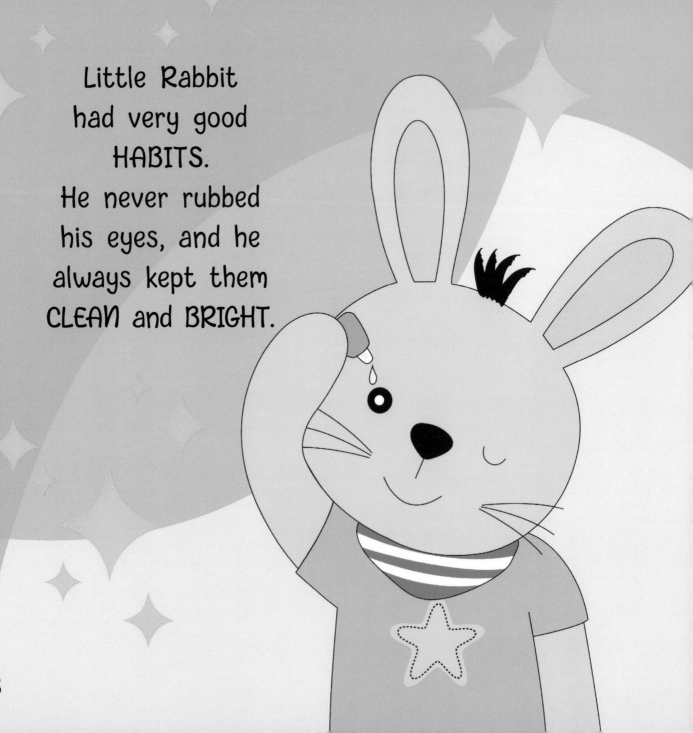

Little Rabbit
had very good
HABITS.
He never rubbed
his eyes, and he
always kept them
CLEAN and BRIGHT.

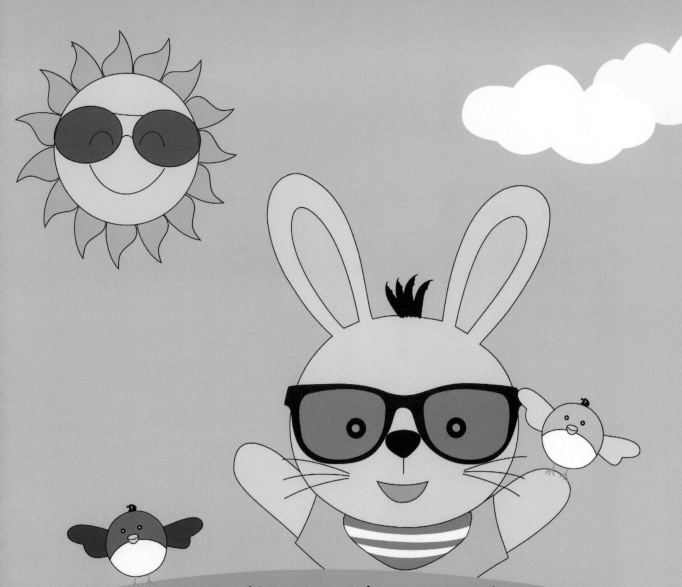

He wore his special
SUNGLASSES on sunny days
at home and at school.

He made sure to read
with proper LIGHTING.

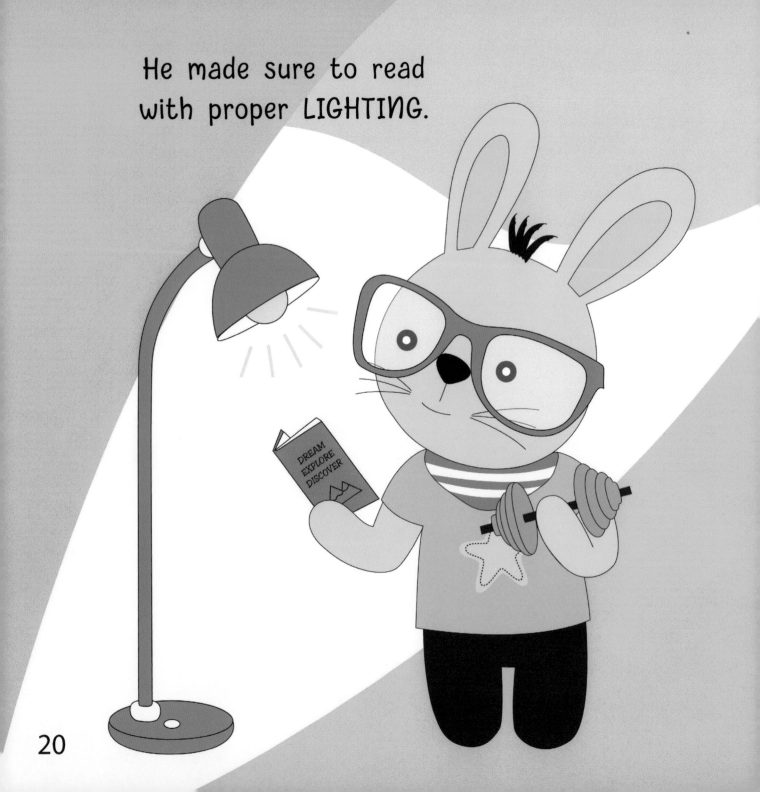

He made sure to eat
HEALTHY FOOD.

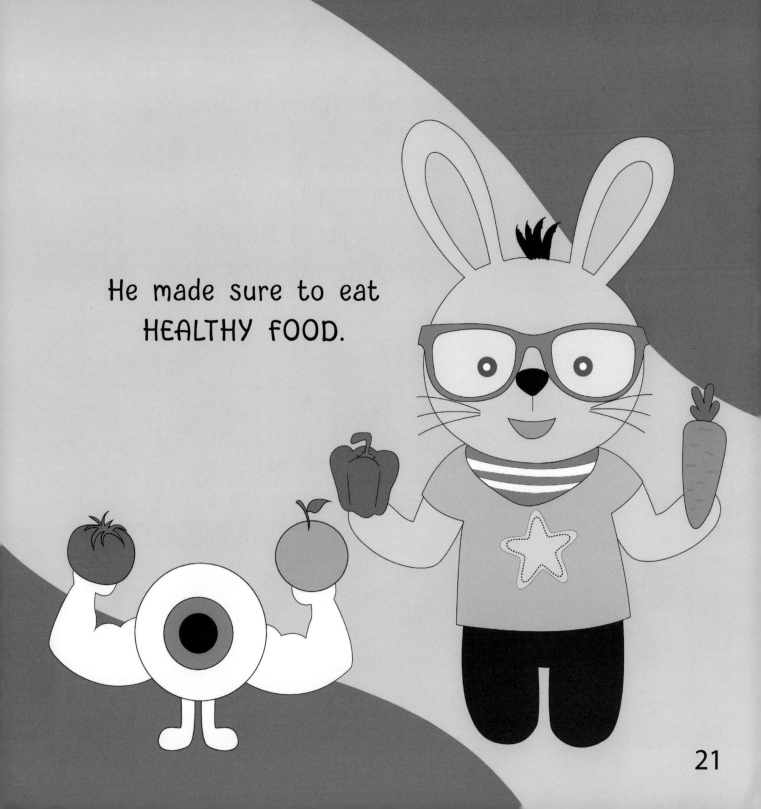

He made sure to get regular
EYE CHECKS with Doctor Bear.

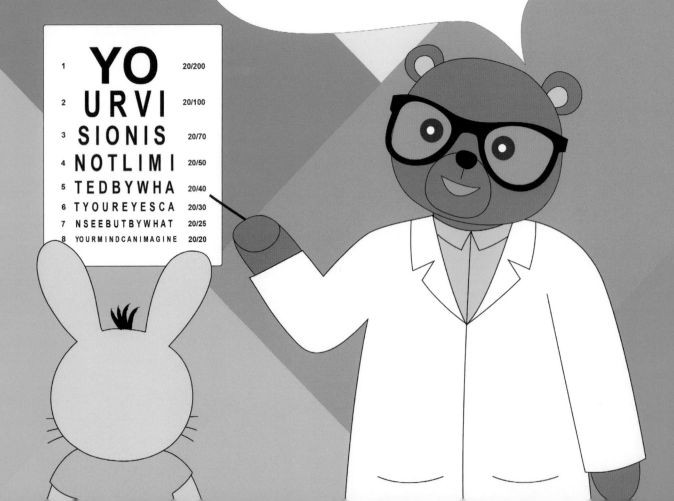

"Remember to give your eyes a BREAK so they can REST."

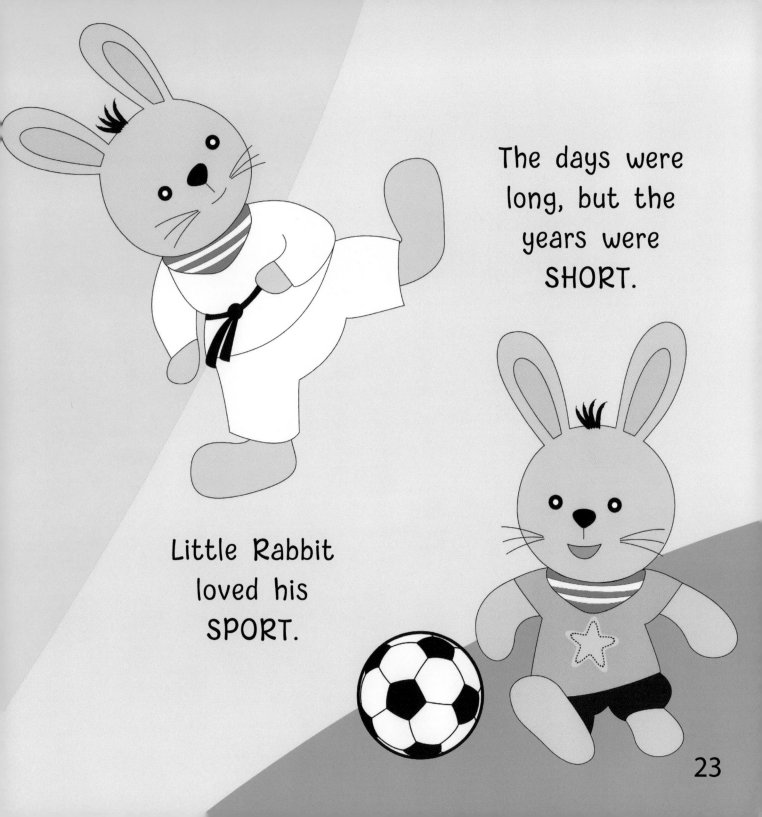

The days were long, but the years were SHORT.

Little Rabbit loved his SPORT.

23

Little Rabbit
stayed SMART
and HEALTHY.

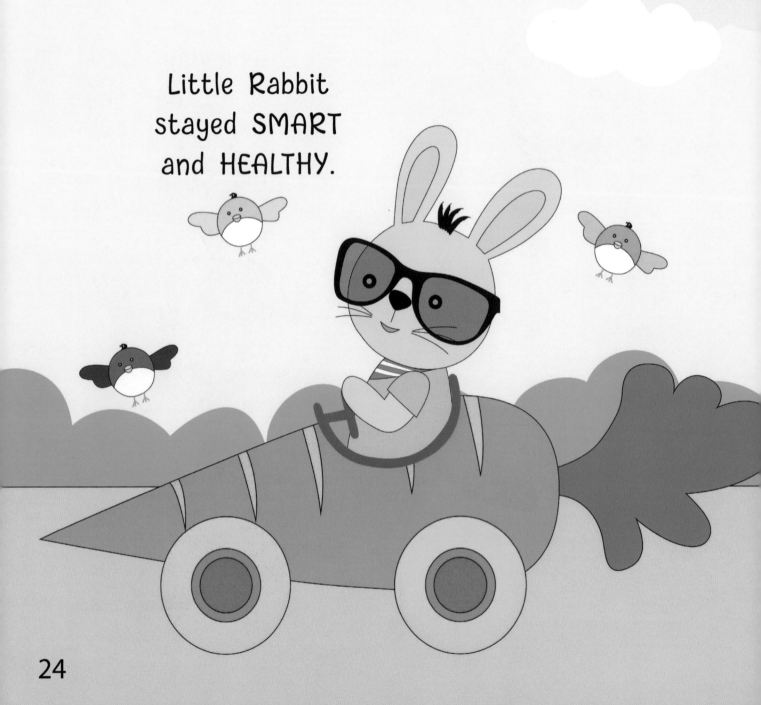

Because he needed his eyes to be strong for the JOURNEY.

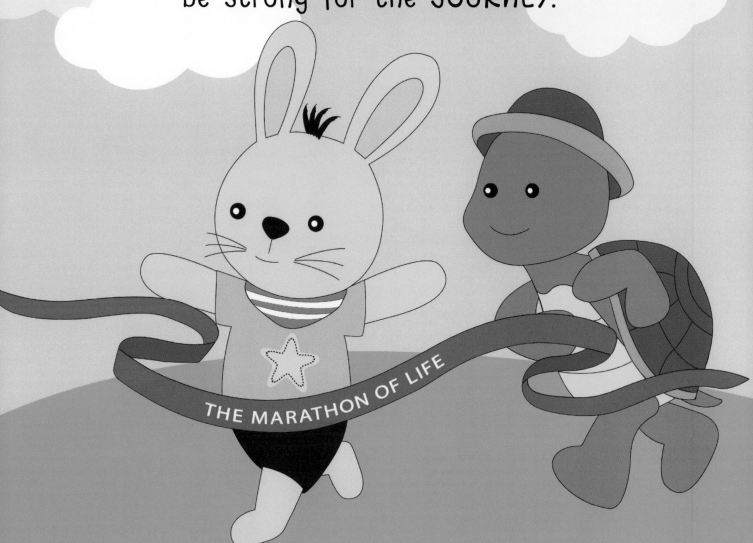

THE MARATHON OF LIFE

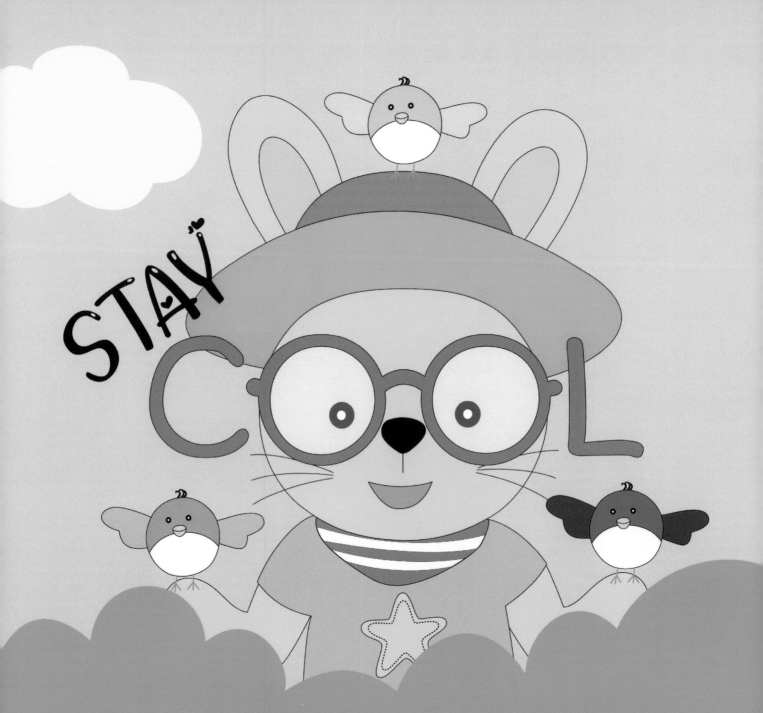

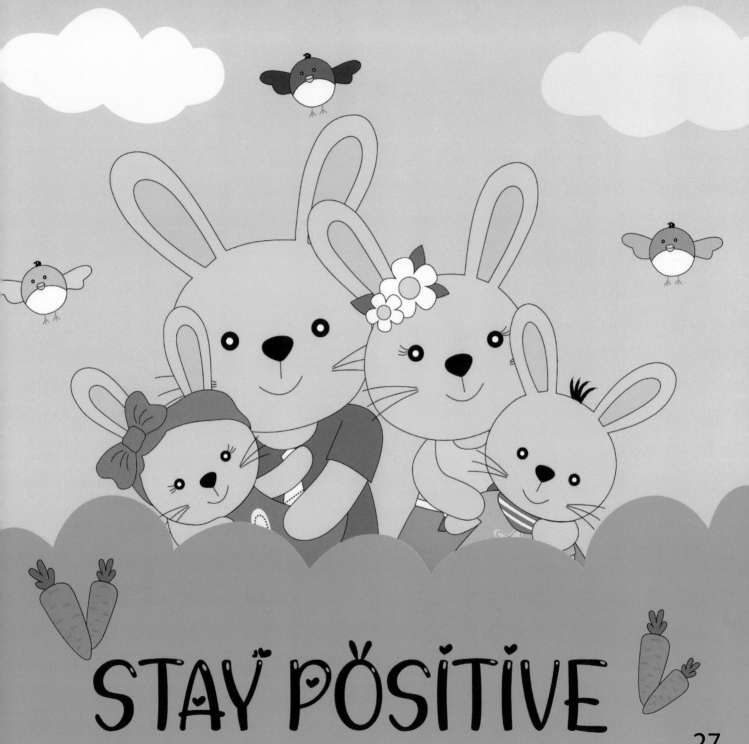

STAY POSITIVE

27

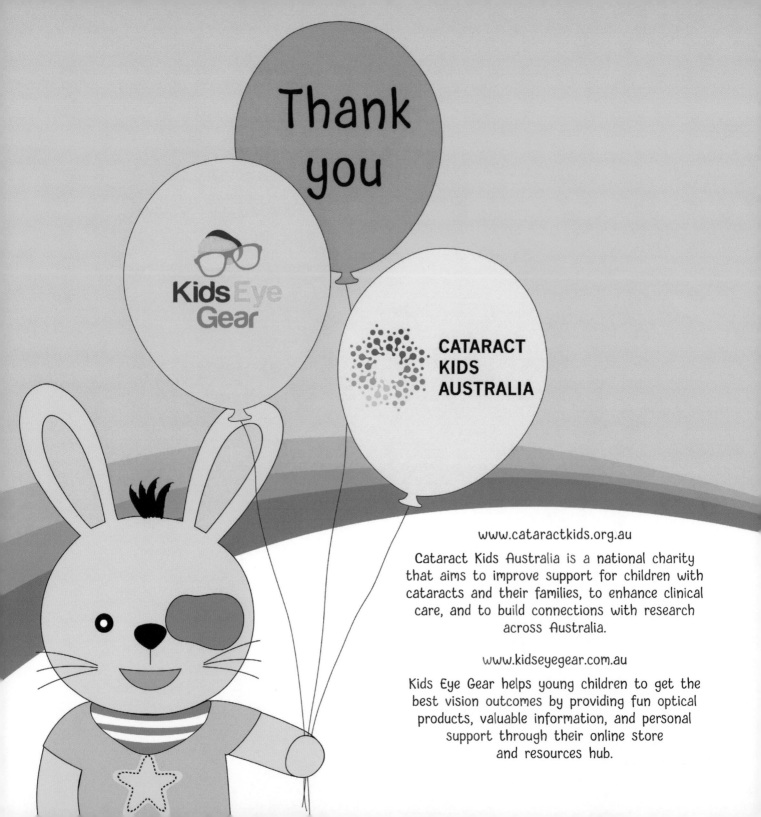

Thank you

Kids Eye Gear

CATARACT KIDS AUSTRALIA

www.cataractkids.org.au

Cataract Kids Australia is a national charity that aims to improve support for children with cataracts and their families, to enhance clinical care, and to build connections with research across Australia.

www.kidseyegear.com.au

Kids Eye Gear helps young children to get the best vision outcomes by providing fun optical products, valuable information, and personal support through their online store and resources hub.

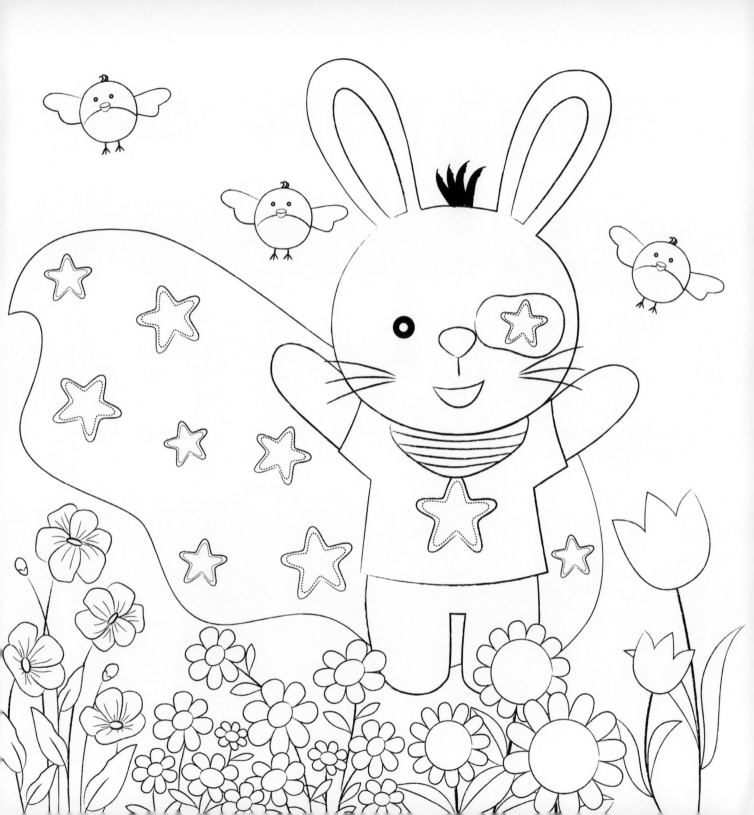

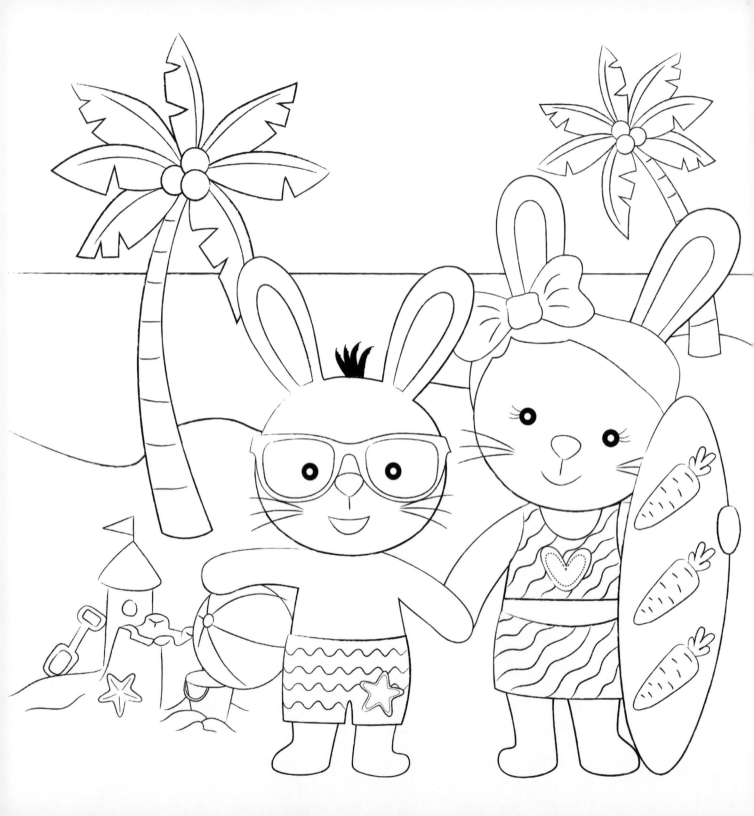

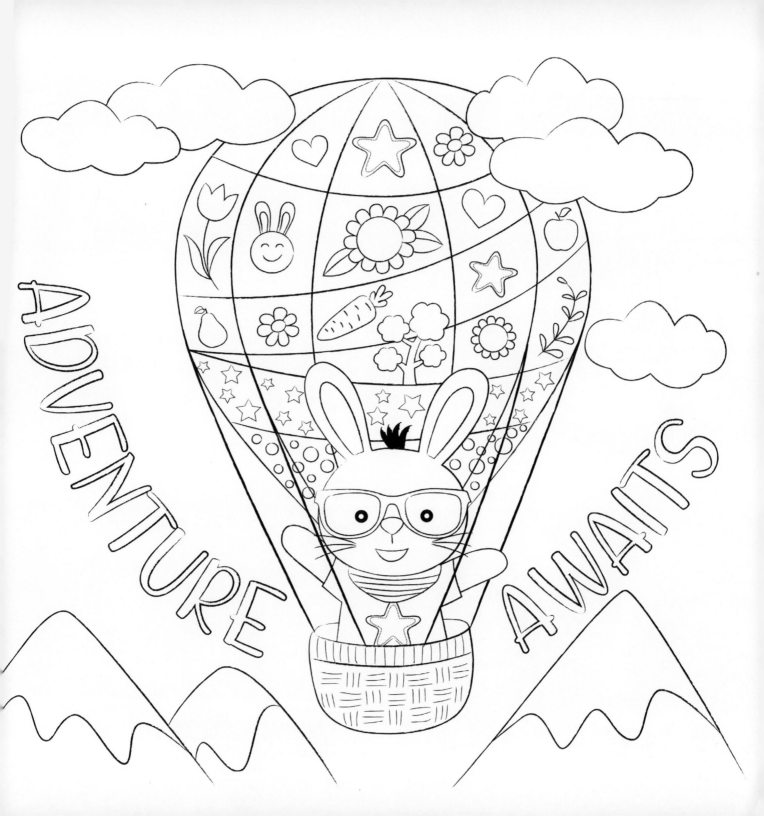

Printed in Great Britain
by Amazon

23917667R00021